OZEMPIC

KNOWLEDGE AND CREATIVITY REGARDING WELLNESS AND CONTROLLING TYPE 2 DIABETES

DR MARY WILLIAMS

TABLE OF CONTENTS

INTRODUCTION

Ozempic, scientifically known as semaglutide, is a groundbreaking medication in the realm of diabetes management. Developed and manufactured by Novo Nordisk, this injectable glucagon-like peptide-1 receptor agonist (GLP-1 RA) has garnered significant attention for its efficacy in improving glycemic control among individuals with type 2 diabetes mellitus. Introduced as a once-weekly subcutaneous injection, Ozempic has emerged as a pivotal therapeutic option, offering patients a convenient and effective means to address the complexities of managing their diabetes.

The advent of Ozempic marks a significant stride in the evolution of diabetes treatment. Semaglutide, the active component of Ozempic, mimics the action of the endogenous GLP-1 hormone, playing a crucial role in regulating glucose homeostasis. This innovative medication not only aids in lowering blood sugar levels but also demonstrates additional benefits such as weight management and cardiovascular risk reduction.

Beyond its physiological impact, Ozempic has reshaped the landscape of patient care by providing a novel approach to diabetes management. Healthcare professionals across the globe have incorporated Ozempic into their armamentarium, considering its favorable efficacy profile and the potential to positively influence patients' overall well-being. As a result, Ozempic has become an integral component in the comprehensive strategy to address the multifaceted challenges associated with type 2 diabetes.

This introduction merely scratches the surface of Ozempic's significance in the context of diabetes care. Subsequent sections will delve deeper into its mechanism of action, indications, dosage and administration, as well as various facets that contribute to its role as a transformative agent in the ongoing pursuit of enhanced diabetes treatment modalities.

WHAT IS OZEMPIC?

Ozempic, the brand name for semaglutide, stands as a beacon of innovation in the landscape of diabetes management. Developed by Novo Nordisk, a pharmaceutical industry leader, Ozempic has garnered widespread attention and acclaim for its profound impact on individuals living with type 2 diabetes mellitus. This comprehensive exploration of Ozempic will traverse its historical evolution, intricate pharmacology, therapeutic indications, pivotal clinical trials, and the broader implications of its integration into the intricate tapestry of modern diabetes care.

Historical Evolution:
The journey of Ozempic commences with the pioneering efforts of Novo Nordisk in the realm of diabetes therapeutics. The development of this medication is rooted in a profound understanding of the intricate molecular pathways governing glucose homeostasis. The quest for an optimal treatment for type 2 diabetes spurred the investigation and synthesis of semaglutide, the active ingredient in Ozempic, ultimately leading to its approval by regulatory authorities.

Pharmacology of Semaglutide:
At the heart of Ozempic's efficacy lies semaglutide, a glucagon-like peptide-1 receptor agonist (GLP-1 RA). This class of medications plays a pivotal role in mimicking the action of the endogenous GLP-1

hormone, a key regulator of glucose metabolism. Semaglutide exerts its effects by enhancing insulin secretion, inhibiting glucagon release, slowing gastric emptying, and promoting a sense of satiety.

The once-weekly subcutaneous injection of Ozempic delivers a sustained release of semaglutide, providing continuous therapeutic benefits throughout the treatment period. This unique pharmacokinetic profile distinguishes Ozempic from other diabetes medications, contributing to its efficacy in achieving and maintaining glycemic control.

Therapeutic Indications:
Ozempic has been approved for use in the management of type 2 diabetes mellitus. Its indications extend to individuals who have not achieved adequate glycemic control with diet and exercise alone. As a second-line treatment, Ozempic offers a valuable option for patients requiring additional intervention to regulate their blood glucose levels.

Moreover, Ozempic has demonstrated efficacy in addressing other aspects of type 2 diabetes management. Studies have indicated its positive impact on body weight, making it a compelling choice for individuals with comorbid obesity. Additionally, the cardiovascular benefits associated with Ozempic contribute to its role as a holistic therapeutic approach.

Clinical Trials and Efficacy:
The journey of Ozempic from development to widespread clinical use has been marked by rigorous

testing through a series of clinical trials. These trials have not only affirmed its safety but also highlighted its efficacy in diverse patient populations. Notable trials, such as the SUSTAIN and PIONEER programs, have provided robust evidence supporting the use of Ozempic in achieving and maintaining glycemic control.

In the SUSTAIN trials, Ozempic demonstrated superior reductions in HbA1c levels compared to placebo and other antidiabetic medications. Furthermore, the PIONEER trials showcased its efficacy across different stages of diabetes treatment, establishing Ozempic as a versatile option in the therapeutic armamentarium.

Mechanism of Action:
Semaglutide's mechanism of action is intricately intertwined with the natural physiological pathways regulating glucose metabolism. As a GLP-1 receptor agonist, Ozempic engages with GLP-1 receptors on pancreatic beta cells, stimulating insulin secretion in a glucose-dependent manner. This mechanism not only aids in lowering elevated blood glucose levels but also minimizes the risk of hypoglycemia.
Beyond the pancreas, semaglutide inhibits glucagon secretion from pancreatic alpha cells, further contributing to glucose control. The deceleration of gastric emptying induced by Ozempic adds another layer of efficacy, preventing rapid spikes in postprandial glucose levels. Additionally, the central nervous system plays a role as semaglutide influences satiety centers, contributing to weight management.

Safety and Tolerability:
A critical aspect of any medication is its safety profile. Ozempic has undergone extensive scrutiny, and its safety and tolerability have been well-established. Common side effects include nausea, vomiting, and diarrhea, although these are often transient and diminish with continued use.

Notably, Ozempic has exhibited a favorable cardiovascular safety profile, a crucial consideration in diabetes management. The SUSTAIN-6 trial demonstrated a reduction in major adverse cardiovascular events in patients treated with Ozempic compared to placebo, reaffirming its cardiovascular benefits.

Practical Considerations:
The administration of Ozempic involves a once-weekly subcutaneous injection, offering a convenient dosing regimen for patients. The availability of pre-filled pens simplifies the administration process, enhancing patient adherence.

Healthcare providers play a pivotal role in guiding patients through the initiation and titration of Ozempic. Education regarding injection techniques, potential side effects, and the importance of regular follow-ups contributes to a collaborative approach in achieving optimal treatment outcomes.

Integration into Diabetes Care:

Ozempic's integration into the broader framework of diabetes care represents a paradigm shift in the approach to managing this complex condition. As a versatile and effective therapeutic option, Ozempic not only addresses glycemic control but also extends its impact to weight management and cardiovascular risk reduction.

The personalized nature of diabetes care underscores the significance of tailoring treatment plans to individual patient needs. Ozempic's inclusion in the arsenal of available medications provides healthcare providers with a valuable tool to optimize treatment strategies and enhance overall patient well-being.

Future Directions:
As research in diabetes therapeutics continues to evolve, the future holds promise for further advancements in GLP-1 receptor agonists. Ongoing investigations may uncover new insights into the nuanced mechanisms of action of Ozempic, potentially expanding its indications or refining its use in specific patient populations.

The continued exploration of combination therapies and the integration of Ozempic into evolving treatment algorithms exemplify the dynamic nature of diabetes care. Collaborative efforts between pharmaceutical researchers, healthcare providers, and patients will shape the trajectory of diabetes management, with Ozempic playing a pivotal role in this ongoing narrative.

Ozempic emerges as a beacon of hope and innovation in the dynamic landscape of diabetes care. Its evolution from conception to widespread clinical use underscores the dedication to improving the lives of individuals affected by type 2 diabetes mellitus. With its unique pharmacology, proven efficacy, and comprehensive benefits beyond glycemic control, Ozempic stands as a testament to the relentless pursuit of excellence in diabetes therapeutics. As we navigate the complexities of this ever-evolving field, Ozempic remains a cornerstone in the holistic approach to managing type 2 diabetes, reshaping the narrative of what is possible in the quest for optimal patient outcomes.

MECHANISM OF ACTION

The mechanism of action of Ozempic (semaglutide) is a fascinating exploration into the intricate physiological pathways that govern glucose homeostasis. As a glucagon-like peptide-1 receptor agonist (GLP-1 RA), semaglutide mimics the action of the endogenous GLP-1 hormone, playing a pivotal role in regulating blood glucose levels. This extensive exploration will delve into the molecular intricacies of Ozempic's mechanism of action, encompassing its interactions with GLP-1 receptors, effects on insulin and glucagon secretion, modulation of gastric emptying, and its impact on satiety centers within the central nervous system.

GLP-1 Receptor Agonism:
The foundation of Ozempic's mechanism of action lies in its agonistic activity at GLP-1 receptors. GLP-1 is a naturally occurring hormone produced by the L-cells of the small intestine in response to nutrient ingestion, primarily carbohydrates. Upon its release into the bloodstream, GLP-1 exerts multifaceted effects on various organs involved in glucose metabolism.
Semaglutide, being a synthetic analog of GLP-1, selectively binds to and activates GLP-1 receptors on pancreatic beta cells, where insulin is produced. This interaction triggers a cascade of intracellular events leading to increased intracellular cyclic AMP (cAMP) levels. Elevated cAMP levels, in turn, stimulate the release of insulin in a glucose-dependent manner. This

unique feature ensures that Ozempic-induced insulin secretion occurs predominantly in response to elevated blood glucose levels, minimizing the risk of hypoglycemia.

Insulin Secretion:
Ozempic's influence on insulin secretion is a pivotal aspect of its therapeutic effect. The stimulation of insulin release by pancreatic beta cells is critical for enhancing glucose uptake by peripheral tissues, such as skeletal muscle and adipose tissue. By facilitating this process, Ozempic helps to lower elevated blood glucose levels, a hallmark of type 2 diabetes.

Moreover, the glucose-dependent nature of Ozempic's insulinotropic effect distinguishes it from some other antidiabetic medications. This property aligns with the physiological regulation of insulin secretion, contributing to a more nuanced and controlled approach to glycemic management.

Inhibition of Glucagon Secretion:
Beyond its effects on insulin, Ozempic exerts a suppressive influence on the secretion of glucagon, the hormone produced by pancreatic alpha cells. Glucagon functions in opposition to insulin, stimulating the liver to release glucose into the bloodstream. In individuals with type 2 diabetes, dysregulated glucagon secretion contributes to elevated fasting and postprandial glucose levels.

Ozempic's ability to inhibit glucagon secretion helps restore the balance between insulin and glucagon, contributing to improved glycemic control. This dual action on both insulin and glucagon provides a comprehensive approach to addressing the underlying pathophysiology of type 2 diabetes.

Gastric Emptying Modulation:
Semaglutide's impact extends beyond the pancreas to the gastrointestinal tract, where it slows gastric emptying. Postprandial hyperglycemia is a common challenge in individuals with diabetes, and the rate at which the stomach empties its contents can influence the post-meal rise in blood glucose levels.
Ozempic's deceleration of gastric emptying contributes to the attenuation of postprandial glucose excursions. By delaying the absorption of nutrients from the gastrointestinal tract, semaglutide helps to mitigate the rapid spikes in blood glucose levels following meals. This effect adds another layer to Ozempic's comprehensive approach to glycemic management.

Satiety Centers in the Central Nervous System:
The intricate interplay between Ozempic and the central nervous system (CNS) constitutes a crucial aspect of its mechanism of action. GLP-1 receptors are distributed in various regions of the CNS, including the hypothalamus, which plays a central role in appetite regulation and satiety.
Semaglutide's activation of GLP-1 receptors in the CNS contributes to its effects on appetite control. By modulating satiety centers, Ozempic induces a sense of fullness and satisfaction, potentially leading to reduced

food intake. This aspect of its mechanism aligns with the broader implications of Ozempic in weight management, an added benefit for individuals with comorbid obesity.

The Integrated Impact:
The convergence of Ozempic's actions on insulin secretion, glucagon inhibition, gastric emptying, and appetite regulation creates a synergistic and integrated impact on glucose metabolism. This multifaceted approach distinguishes GLP-1 receptor agonists, including Ozempic, as a unique class of medications in the diabetes treatment landscape.

The comprehensive modulation of various components of glucose homeostasis positions Ozempic as a valuable therapeutic option for individuals with type 2 diabetes. Its ability to address multiple facets of the underlying pathophysiology contributes to its efficacy in achieving and maintaining glycemic control, making it a cornerstone in the management of this complex condition.

Considerations for Individualization:
While Ozempic's mechanism of action provides a robust foundation for its therapeutic efficacy, the individualization of treatment remains paramount in diabetes care. Patient-specific factors, including comorbidities, lifestyle, and preferences, influence the selection and optimization of therapeutic regimens.

Healthcare providers play a crucial role in tailoring treatment plans to meet the unique needs of each patient. The nuanced understanding of Ozempic's mechanism of action empowers providers to make informed decisions, optimizing its integration into individualized diabetes management strategies.

Safety and Tolerability:
Understanding the intricacies of Ozempic's mechanism of action is incomplete without acknowledging its safety profile. Like any medication, Ozempic is associated with potential side effects. Nausea, vomiting, and diarrhea are among the common adverse events reported, particularly during the initial phases of treatment. However, these side effects are generally transient and tend to diminish with continued use.

Moreover, Ozempic has undergone rigorous evaluation, including cardiovascular outcomes trials, to assess its safety in individuals with diabetes. The SUSTAIN-6 trial demonstrated a reduction in major adverse cardiovascular events in patients treated with Ozempic compared to placebo, further supporting its cardiovascular safety.

Future Directions and Evolving Understanding:
As the landscape of diabetes research advances, the exploration of GLP-1 receptor agonists and their mechanisms of action continues to evolve. Ongoing investigations seek to uncover additional insights into the nuanced interactions between Ozempic and the various components of glucose metabolism.

Future research endeavors may unveil novel applications for Ozempic beyond its current indications. The potential expansion of its use in specific patient populations or the exploration of combination therapies represents exciting avenues for further exploration. The dynamic nature of diabetes care underscores the importance of staying abreast of emerging research findings to continually refine and enhance treatment approaches.

Ozempic's mechanism of action is a symphony of intricate molecular events that harmonize to restore balance in glucose homeostasis. Its role as a GLP-1 receptor agonist encompasses not only insulinotropic effects but also the inhibition of glucagon, modulation of gastric emptying, and the modulation of satiety centers in the CNS. This multifaceted approach positions Ozempic as a cornerstone in the management of type 2 diabetes, offering a comprehensive and integrated solution to the complex challenges posed by this condition.

INDICATIONS

The indications for Ozempic (semaglutide) encompass a comprehensive understanding of its therapeutic role in the management of type 2 diabetes mellitus. As a glucagon-like peptide-1 receptor agonist (GLP-1 RA), Ozempic has demonstrated efficacy in diverse patient populations, offering a multifaceted approach to address the complex pathophysiology of this prevalent metabolic disorder. This extensive exploration will traverse the indications for Ozempic, including its role as a second-line treatment, considerations for initiation, and its potential benefits beyond glycemic control.

Indications:
Ozempic is indicated for use in adults with type 2 diabetes mellitus to improve glycemic control. This recommendation extends to individuals who have not achieved adequate blood glucose regulation through diet and exercise alone. Positioned as a second-line treatment, Ozempic provides an additional therapeutic option for patients requiring intervention beyond lifestyle modifications or first-line oral antidiabetic medications.
The indications for Ozempic have evolved as a result of rigorous clinical trials, which have not only affirmed its efficacy but also illuminated its broader impact on various aspects of diabetes management. From glycemic control to cardiovascular benefits and weight management, Ozempic's indications reflect a

comprehensive approach to addressing the multifaceted challenges associated with type 2 diabetes.

Second-Line Treatment:
The placement of Ozempic as a second-line treatment underscores its role in the continuum of diabetes care. As type 2 diabetes progresses, the need for interventions that target multiple aspects of glucose metabolism becomes increasingly critical. While lifestyle modifications and oral antidiabetic medications may suffice in the early stages, the addition of injectable therapies like Ozempic becomes pivotal in achieving and maintaining optimal glycemic control.

Healthcare providers often initiate Ozempic when first-line treatments, such as metformin, fail to adequately manage blood glucose levels. The decision to transition to Ozempic is informed by individual patient factors, including disease severity, comorbidities, and the overall treatment plan tailored to the patient's unique needs.

Considerations for Initiation:
Initiating Ozempic involves a careful assessment of patient-specific factors and consideration of the broader treatment strategy. Healthcare providers play a central role in guiding this process, taking into account the patient's medical history, current medications, and treatment goals.

Common considerations for initiating Ozempic include:

Inadequate Glycemic Control: Ozempic is often initiated when blood glucose levels remain elevated despite adherence to lifestyle modifications and oral antidiabetic medications. The goal is to achieve and maintain target HbA1c levels, minimizing the risk of long-term complications associated with uncontrolled diabetes.

Weight Management Goals: The potential for weight loss with Ozempic makes it a favorable choice for individuals with type 2 diabetes and comorbid obesity. Providers may consider Ozempic in patients where weight management is a significant therapeutic goal.

Cardiovascular Risk Reduction: The cardiovascular benefits associated with Ozempic, as demonstrated in clinical trials, contribute to its consideration in patients with established cardiovascular disease or those at risk. Cardiovascular outcomes trials, such as SUSTAIN-6, have shown a reduction in major adverse cardiovascular events with Ozempic.

Patient Preferences and Lifestyle: The once-weekly dosing regimen of Ozempic, administered via subcutaneous injection, may align well with the lifestyle and preferences of certain patients. Education and communication play a crucial role in addressing any potential concerns or misconceptions regarding injectable therapies.

Comprehensive Glycemic Control:

Ozempic's primary indication revolves around its ability to improve glycemic control in individuals with type 2 diabetes. By acting as a GLP-1 receptor agonist, Ozempic addresses the underlying insulin resistance and dysregulation of insulin secretion characteristic of type 2 diabetes.

The once-weekly subcutaneous injection of Ozempic provides sustained GLP-1 receptor agonism, offering a continuous therapeutic effect throughout the treatment period. This approach contrasts with the more frequent dosing required for some other antidiabetic medications, contributing to enhanced patient adherence and convenience.

Clinical trials, including the SUSTAIN and PIONEER programs, have consistently demonstrated Ozempic's efficacy in reducing HbA1c levels. The robust reductions observed in these trials underscore its role as a potent tool in achieving and maintaining optimal glycemic control.

Cardiovascular Benefits:
Ozempic's indications extend beyond glycemic control to encompass cardiovascular risk reduction. Cardiovascular outcomes trials, such as SUSTAIN-6, have investigated the impact of Ozempic on major adverse cardiovascular events in patients with type 2 diabetes and established cardiovascular disease.

The results of these trials have shown a significant reduction in the risk of major adverse cardiovascular events, including cardiovascular death, non-fatal myocardial infarction, and non-fatal stroke, in individuals treated with Ozempic. This cardiovascular benefit enhances the overall appeal of Ozempic as a therapeutic option for individuals with type 2 diabetes, especially those with a heightened cardiovascular risk.

Weight Management:
A notable feature that distinguishes Ozempic is its impact on body weight. Individuals with type 2 diabetes often face challenges related to weight gain or obesity, which can exacerbate insulin resistance and complicate overall disease management.
Ozempic's ability to induce weight loss makes it particularly attractive for individuals with comorbid obesity. Clinical trials have demonstrated significant reductions in body weight in patients treated with Ozempic, further positioning it as a valuable tool in the comprehensive management of type 2 diabetes.

Patient-Centric Approach:
The indications for Ozempic underscore the importance of a patient-centric approach in diabetes care. Individualized treatment plans that consider the unique needs, preferences, and goals of each patient are essential for optimizing therapeutic outcomes.
Healthcare providers collaborate with patients to establish realistic treatment goals, addressing not only glycemic control but also factors such as weight management and cardiovascular risk. Shared decision-making and ongoing communication between providers and patients contribute to a collaborative and effective approach to diabetes management.

Special Populations:
Ozempic's indications extend to specific populations within the broader spectrum of type 2 diabetes. While generally indicated for adults, considerations may arise in special populations, such as:

Elderly Patients: Healthcare providers may consider the individualized needs and potential comorbidities of elderly patients when prescribing Ozempic. Close monitoring and adjustment of treatment plans based on age-related factors are essential.

Patients with Renal Impairment: Ozempic has been studied in patients with varying degrees of renal impairment. Providers may adjust the dosage based on renal function, ensuring that the benefits of Ozempic are optimized while minimizing the risk of adverse effects.

Pediatric Population: As of the knowledge cutoff date in January 2022, Ozempic's indications are primarily focused on adults. The safety and efficacy of Ozempic in pediatric populations are areas of ongoing research.

The indications for Ozempic encapsulate its pivotal role in the dynamic landscape of type 2 diabetes management. From its position as a second-line treatment to its broader impact on cardiovascular risk reduction and weight management, Ozempic represents a versatile and effective therapeutic option. As healthcare providers navigate the complexities of diabetes care, the indications for Ozempic guide the thoughtful integration of this GLP-1 receptor agonist into individualized treatment plans, ultimately contributing to the holistic well-being of individuals living with type 2 diabetes mellitus.

DOSAGE AND ADMINISTRATION

The dosage and administration of Ozempic (semaglutide) play a crucial role in optimizing its therapeutic effects while ensuring patient adherence and safety. As a once-weekly subcutaneous injectable medication, Ozempic offers a convenient dosing regimen for individuals with type 2 diabetes mellitus. This extensive exploration will delve into the nuanced aspects of Ozempic's dosage, including initiation, titration, administration techniques, potential considerations for missed doses, and practical guidance for healthcare providers and patients alike.

Dosage and Administration:
Ozempic is administered as a subcutaneous injection once weekly. The medication is typically supplied in pre-filled pens, simplifying the administration process and enhancing patient convenience. The pre-filled pens are available in various strengths, allowing for flexibility in dosing based on individual patient needs.
The dosage of Ozempic is expressed in milligrams (mg), reflecting the amount of semaglutide delivered with each injection. The initiation and titration of Ozempic are guided by the goal of achieving and maintaining optimal

glycemic control while minimizing the risk of adverse effects.

Initiation of Ozempic:
The initiation of Ozempic involves a thoughtful assessment of the patient's current antidiabetic regimen, glycemic control, and overall treatment goals.

Healthcare providers consider factors such as:

Current Treatment Plan: Ozempic is often initiated as a second-line treatment in individuals with type 2 diabetes who have not achieved adequate glycemic control with diet and exercise alone or with first-line oral antidiabetic medications, such as metformin.

Baseline HbA1c Levels: The patient's baseline HbA1c levels influence the decision to initiate Ozempic and guide the target for glycemic control. Higher baseline HbA1c levels may warrant more aggressive treatment initiation and titration.

Cardiovascular Risk: The cardiovascular benefits associated with Ozempic, as demonstrated in clinical trials, may influence the decision to initiate the medication in individuals with a history of cardiovascular disease or at an increased risk.

Patient Preferences: The once-weekly dosing regimen and availability of pre-filled pens may align with the preferences and lifestyle of certain patients. Patient education regarding the benefits and practical aspects of Ozempic administration contributes to informed decision-making.

Dosage Initiation and Titration:
The initiation and titration of Ozempic involve a gradual approach to optimize glycemic control while minimizing the risk of adverse effects, particularly gastrointestinal symptoms that may occur during the initial phase of treatment.

The typical initiation and titration process includes:

Initial Dose: The standard starting dose of Ozempic is often 0.25 mg once weekly. This lower dose minimizes the risk of gastrointestinal side effects during the initial weeks of treatment.

Titration: After 4 weeks at the initial dose, the dosage is titrated to 0.5 mg once weekly. This incremental approach allows patients to acclimate to the medication while providing a more gradual onset of its effects.

Maintenance Dose: Following the titration phase, the maintenance dose of Ozempic is 1 mg once weekly. This dosage is often effective in achieving and maintaining glycemic control for many patients.
The gradual titration of Ozempic aligns with the pharmacokinetics of semaglutide and supports a well-tolerated introduction to the medication. Individual

patient response, tolerability, and glycemic control guide the decision-making process during titration.

Administration Techniques:
Proper administration techniques are crucial to ensure the efficacy and safety of Ozempic. Healthcare providers play a central role in educating patients on the correct procedures for self-injection.

Key aspects of Ozempic administration include:

Subcutaneous Injection: Ozempic is administered via subcutaneous injection in the thigh, abdomen, or upper arm. The injection site should be rotated to minimize the risk of lipodystrophy or injection site reactions.

Pre-filled Pens: The pre-filled pens come equipped with a needle for injection. Patients should be instructed on the correct handling of the pen, including proper storage, removal of the needle cap, and the injection technique.

Dosing Timing: Ozempic is typically administered on the same day each week. Consistency in dosing timing contributes to a predictable therapeutic effect and aids in patient adherence.

Needle Disposal: Proper disposal of needles and pre-filled pens is essential for patient safety and compliance with disposal regulations. Patients should be provided with clear instructions on safe needle disposal.

Patient Training: Healthcare providers should offer thorough training on injection techniques during the initiation visit and reinforce these instructions during follow-up appointments. Patient understanding and confidence in self-administration contribute to adherence.

Considerations for Missed Doses:
Addressing missed doses is an integral aspect of patient education to maintain the efficacy of

Ozempic Guidelines for managing missed doses include:

Missed Weekly Dose: If a dose is missed, the patient should administer it as soon as possible within 5 days of the missed dose. If more than 5 days have passed, the next dose should be administered on the regularly scheduled day.

Additional Doses: Patients should not administer two doses on the same day to make up for a missed dose. Doubling the dose does not provide additional therapeutic benefits and may increase the risk of adverse effects.

Regular Schedule: Patients should resume their regular once-weekly dosing schedule after a missed dose. Consistency in dosing timing contributes to optimal therapeutic outcomes.

Practical Guidance for Healthcare Providers:
Healthcare providers play a pivotal role in facilitating the successful implementation of Ozempic in the overall diabetes management plan.

Practical guidance for providers includes:

Patient Education: Thoroughly educate patients on the benefits, administration techniques, and potential side effects of Ozempic. Address any concerns or misconceptions to enhance patient understanding and adherence.

Monitoring and Follow-Up: Regular monitoring of blood glucose levels and HbA1c, along with periodic follow-up appointments, allows healthcare providers to assess the patient's response to Ozempic and make any necessary adjustments to the treatment plan.

Individualization of Treatment: Consider individual patient factors, preferences, and treatment goals when initiating and titrating Ozempic. The personalized nature of diabetes care informs decisions regarding the most appropriate dosage and administration strategy for each patient.

Collaborative Decision-Making: Engage in collaborative decision-making with patients, involving them in the treatment plan and considering their preferences and lifestyle. Shared decision-making enhances patient autonomy and adherence.

Adverse Event Management: Provide guidance on managing potential adverse events, such as gastrointestinal symptoms, and educate patients on when to seek medical attention. Addressing adverse events promptly contributes to a positive treatment experience.

Special Populations:
Considerations for dosage and administration may vary in special populations, and healthcare providers should tailor their approach based on individual patient needs.

Key considerations include:

Elderly Patients: Healthcare providers may exercise caution in elderly patients and consider starting at the lower end of the dosing spectrum. Monitoring for potential adverse effects and adjusting the dosage based on individual response is essential.

Renal Impairment: Adjustments in the dosage may be necessary in patients with renal impairment. Monitoring renal function and making dosage adjustments accordingly contribute to the safe use of Ozempic in this population.

SIDE EFFECTS

Exploring the side effects of Ozempic (semaglutide) provides a comprehensive understanding of the potential impact on individuals using this glucagon-like peptide-1 receptor agonist (GLP-1 RA) for the management of type 2 diabetes mellitus. While Ozempic has demonstrated efficacy in improving glycemic control, its use is associated with specific side effects that warrant consideration. This extensive exploration will delve into the various side effects of Ozempic, including both common and rare occurrences, gastrointestinal symptoms, potential cardiovascular implications, and considerations for special populations.

Side Effects:
As with any medication, Ozempic has a range of potential side effects that may vary in frequency and severity among individuals. It's essential for healthcare providers and patients to be aware of these side effects to facilitate informed decision-making, monitoring, and timely management. Common side effects of Ozempic include gastrointestinal symptoms, while less common side effects and serious adverse events are also discussed below.

Common Side Effects:

Gastrointestinal Symptoms:

Nausea: One of the most commonly reported side effects of Ozempic is nausea. Patients initiating treatment may experience mild to moderate nausea, particularly during the initial weeks of therapy. In most cases, this symptom tends to diminish over time.

Vomiting: Some individuals may experience vomiting, which is often transient and occurs more frequently during the early stages of treatment. Patients are advised to consult their healthcare providers if vomiting persists or becomes severe.

Diarrhea: Diarrhea is another gastrointestinal symptom associated with Ozempic use. Like nausea and vomiting, diarrhea tends to be more prevalent during the initial weeks of treatment and often improves with continued use.

These gastrointestinal symptoms are generally mild to moderate in severity and typically subside as patients acclimate to Ozempic. Providers should educate patients on the transient nature of these side effects and offer guidance on managing symptoms, such as taking Ozempic with meals to potentially mitigate gastrointestinal discomfort.

Less Common Side Effects:
While less common, some individuals may experience side effects beyond gastrointestinal symptoms. These include:

Hypoglycemia: While Ozempic itself does not typically cause hypoglycemia when used as a monotherapy, the risk of hypoglycemia may increase when Ozempic is combined with other antidiabetic medications, especially those that can cause low blood sugar.

Headache: Headache is reported less frequently but may occur in some individuals. It is usually mild and transient.

Fatigue: Fatigue or tiredness is a less common side effect that may be experienced by some individuals using Ozempic.

Injection Site Reactions: Localized reactions at the injection site, such as redness or swelling, can occur but are generally mild.
Providers should be vigilant in monitoring patients for these less common side effects, especially when initiating or adjusting the dosage of Ozempic. Patient education regarding potential side effects and their management is crucial to enhance adherence and mitigate concerns.

Serious Adverse Events:
While uncommon, serious adverse events associated with Ozempic use include:

Pancreatitis: There have been rare reports of pancreatitis in individuals using GLP-1 receptor agonists, including Ozempic. Providers should be cautious in patients with a history of pancreatitis, and prompt evaluation is warranted if symptoms such as persistent severe abdominal pain occur.

Hypersensitivity Reactions: Hypersensitivity reactions, including severe allergic reactions (anaphylaxis), may occur. Providers should educate patients about the signs of hypersensitivity and advise them to seek immediate medical attention if such reactions occur.

Acute Kidney Injury: Cases of acute kidney injury, often reversible upon discontinuation of the medication, have been reported. Providers should assess renal function before initiating Ozempic and monitor patients for changes in renal function during treatment.

Thyroid C-Cell Tumors: GLP-1 receptor agonists, including Ozempic, have been associated with an increased risk of thyroid C-cell tumors in animal studies. However, the relevance of this finding to humans remains uncertain. Routine monitoring of thyroid function is recommended.

Cardiovascular Implications:
A notable aspect of Ozempic's safety profile is its cardiovascular outcomes trial, SUSTAIN-6, which demonstrated a reduction in major adverse cardiovascular events in individuals treated with Ozempic compared to placebo. The trial included a diverse population of patients with type 2 diabetes and

established cardiovascular disease or at high cardiovascular risk.

Ozempic's cardiovascular benefits, including a reduction in cardiovascular death, non-fatal myocardial infarction, and non-fatal stroke, contribute to its appeal as a therapeutic option for individuals with type 2 diabetes and cardiovascular comorbidities.

Considerations for Special Populations:
Understanding the side effect profile of Ozempic in special populations is essential for tailoring treatment plans. Considerations include:

Elderly Patients: Elderly patients may be more susceptible to certain side effects, such as gastrointestinal symptoms. Providers should exercise caution and closely monitor for adverse events, adjusting the dosage if necessary.

Renal Impairment: Individuals with renal impairment may require dosage adjustments, as Ozempic is primarily excreted through the renal route. Regular monitoring of renal function is essential in this population.

Pediatric Population: As of the knowledge cutoff date in January 2022, the safety and efficacy of Ozempic in the pediatric population have not been extensively studied. The use of Ozempic in children and adolescents should be approached with caution, and decisions should be based on individual patient needs.

Practical Guidance for Healthcare Providers:

Patient Education: Thoroughly educate patients on the potential side effects of Ozempic, emphasizing the transient nature of common gastrointestinal symptoms and the importance of reporting any persistent or severe symptoms.

Monitoring and Follow-Up: Implement a structured monitoring plan, including regular assessments of glycemic control, renal function, and cardiovascular risk factors. Periodic follow-up appointments allow providers to address any emerging concerns and optimize the treatment plan.

Adherence Support: Support patient adherence by providing practical guidance on medication administration, including injection techniques and dosing schedules. Addressing any concerns or misconceptions about potential side effects enhances patient confidence in the treatment.

Individualization of Treatment: Individualize treatment plans based on patient-specific factors, including comorbidities, preferences, and treatment goals. Consideration of special populations and potential contraindications guides decision-making.

Collaborative Decision-Making: Engage in collaborative decision-making with patients, involving them in discussions about potential side effects and the overall management plan. Shared decision-making enhances patient autonomy and fosters a collaborative approach to care.

Understanding the side effects of Ozempic is integral to the safe and effective management of type 2 diabetes. While common gastrointestinal symptoms are often transient and manageable, providers must remain vigilant for less common side effects and serious adverse events. The cardiovascular benefits associated with Ozempic contribute to its appeal, especially in individuals with cardiovascular comorbidities. Practical guidance, individualized treatment plans, and ongoing monitoring enhance patient safety and optimize the overall therapeutic experience with Ozempic.

CONTRAINDICATIONS

Contraindications are essential considerations in the prescription and administration of medications, guiding healthcare providers in identifying situations where the use of a particular drug may pose risks or be inappropriate for a specific individual. Ozempic (semaglutide), a glucagon-like peptide-1 receptor agonist (GLP-1 RA) used in the management of type 2 diabetes mellitus, is subject to specific contraindications that necessitate careful evaluation and decision-making by healthcare professionals. This extensive exploration will delve into the contraindications associated with Ozempic, covering general contraindications, special populations, and situations that warrant caution or adjustments in treatment plans.

General Contraindications:

Hypersensitivity to Semaglutide or Components:

Ozempic should not be prescribed to individuals with a known hypersensitivity or allergic reaction to semaglutide or any of its components. Hypersensitivity reactions can manifest as severe allergic reactions, including anaphylaxis, which require immediate medical attention.

Personal or Family History of Medullary Thyroid Carcinoma (MTC):

Ozempic is contraindicated in individuals with a personal or family history of medullary thyroid carcinoma (MTC) or in patients with Multiple Endocrine Neoplasia syndrome type 2 (MEN 2). GLP-1 receptor agonists, including Ozempic, have been associated with an increased risk of MTC based on preclinical studies.

Prior Serious Hypersensitivity Reaction to GLP-1 Receptor Agonists:

Individuals who have experienced a serious hypersensitivity reaction, including anaphylaxis, to other GLP-1 receptor agonists should not use Ozempic. Cross-reactivity between different GLP-1 receptor agonists may occur, and caution is warranted in such cases.

Cardiovascular Considerations:
While Ozempic has demonstrated cardiovascular benefits in clinical trials, specific considerations and contraindications exist for certain cardiovascular situations:

Heart Failure:

Ozempic is contraindicated in individuals with a history of heart failure. The cardiovascular outcomes trial, SUSTAIN-6, demonstrated a reduction in major adverse cardiovascular events with Ozempic, but caution is advised in patients with heart failure, especially those with severe or unstable heart failure.

Chronic Kidney Disease:

Ozempic's safety in individuals with advanced chronic kidney disease (CKD) has not been extensively studied. Given that GLP-1 receptor agonists, in general, may affect renal function, caution is advised in patients with severe renal impairment or end-stage renal disease.

Gastrointestinal Conditions:

Gastroparesis:

Individuals with gastroparesis, a condition characterized by delayed gastric emptying, may be at an increased risk of gastrointestinal adverse effects with Ozempic. Caution is warranted, and the potential risks and benefits should be carefully evaluated before prescribing Ozempic in these patients.

Inflammatory Bowel Disease:

Inflammatory bowel disease (IBD), including Crohn's disease and ulcerative colitis, may be associated with an increased risk of gastrointestinal adverse events. Healthcare providers should exercise caution when considering Ozempic in individuals with a history of IBD.

Endocrine Conditions:
Personal or Family History of Multiple Endocrine

Neoplasia Syndrome Type 2 (MEN 2):

Ozempic is contraindicated in individuals with a personal or family history of MEN 2. This genetic disorder is associated with an increased risk of medullary thyroid carcinoma (MTC), a rare type of thyroid cancer.

Prior Pancreatitis:

Individuals with a history of pancreatitis should not use Ozempic. Pancreatitis has been reported with GLP-1 receptor agonists, and caution is warranted in individuals with a history of this condition.

Special Populations:

Pregnancy and Breastfeeding:

The safety of Ozempic during pregnancy and breastfeeding has not been established. Ozempic should only be used during pregnancy if the potential benefits justify the potential risks to the fetus. It is not known whether Ozempic is excreted in human breast milk.

Pediatric Population:

Ozempic is not indicated for use in children and adolescents. The safety and efficacy of Ozempic in the pediatric population have not been established, and its use in this age group is not recommended.

Elderly Population:

While Ozempic can be used in elderly individuals, caution is advised, especially in those with comorbidities or conditions that may increase the risk of adverse events. Dosage adjustments and close monitoring may be necessary.

Considerations for Special Situations:

Surgery and Acute Illness:

During periods of acute illness or major surgery, the use of Ozempic may be temporarily discontinued. Individuals may require alternative means of glycemic control during these situations.

Renal Impairment:

Ozempic is primarily excreted through the renal route. In patients with renal impairment, adjustments to the dosage of Ozempic may be necessary. Close monitoring of renal function is recommended in this population. Dosing Adjustments with Concomitant

Medications:

Concomitant use of medications that affect renal function or require dosage adjustments in renal impairment may necessitate modifications in the dosing regimen of Ozempic. Providers should carefully assess potential drug interactions.

Practical Guidance for Healthcare Providers:

Comprehensive Patient Assessment:

Conduct a thorough patient assessment, including medical history, family history, and a review of current medications, before prescribing Ozempic. This comprehensive evaluation aids in identifying contraindications and potential risks.

Individualized Treatment Plans:

Individualize treatment plans based on patient-specific factors, considering contraindications, comorbidities, and treatment goals. Shared decision-making with patients enhances understanding and collaboration in the management of diabetes.

Regular Monitoring:

Implement a structured monitoring plan, including regular assessments of glycemic control, cardiovascular risk factors, and potential adverse events. Regular follow-up appointments allow for ongoing evaluation and adjustments as needed.

Patient Education:

Thoroughly educate patients on contraindications and potential risks associated with Ozempic. Clear communication enhances patient understanding and facilitates adherence to treatment recommendations.

Collaboration with Specialists:

Collaborate with specialists, such as endocrinologists, cardiologists, and nephrologists, when managing individuals with complex medical conditions or contraindications that require specialized expertise.

Contraindications serve as crucial guidelines in the safe and effective use of Ozempic for individuals with type 2 diabetes mellitus. Healthcare providers must carefully evaluate each patient's medical history, assess potential contraindications, and tailor treatment plans accordingly. By considering contraindications, individualizing treatment, and closely monitoring patients, healthcare professionals contribute to optimizing the overall safety and efficacy of Ozempic in the diverse population of individuals with type 2 diabetes.

DRUG INTERACTIONS

Understanding the potential drug interactions associated with Ozempic (semaglutide) is paramount for healthcare providers to ensure safe and effective management of type 2 diabetes mellitus. Drug interactions can impact the pharmacokinetics and pharmacodynamics of Ozempic, potentially influencing its efficacy and safety. This extensive exploration will delve into the various drug interactions associated with Ozempic, covering interactions with other antidiabetic medications, drugs affecting renal function, gastrointestinal motility, and those requiring dosage adjustments when used concomitantly with Ozempic.

Interaction with Antidiabetic Medications:

Insulin and Insulin Secretagogues:

Combining Ozempic with insulin or insulin secretagogues (e.g., sulfonylureas) may increase the risk of hypoglycemia. Providers should carefully adjust insulin or secretagogue doses when initiating Ozempic to minimize the potential for low blood sugar. Regular monitoring of blood glucose levels is essential during the titration phase.

Dipeptidyl Peptidase-4 (DPP-4) Inhibitors:

Ozempic can be used concomitantly with DPP-4 inhibitors, but caution is advised. While combining these medications is generally well-tolerated, providers should monitor for potential additive effects on glycemic control and adjust doses as needed.

Sodium-Glucose Co-Transporter 2 (SGLT2) Inhibitors:

Ozempic can be used with SGLT2 inhibitors, offering a complementary approach to managing hyperglycemia. However, providers should monitor for potential additive effects on renal function and the risk of dehydration. Adjustments in SGLT2 inhibitor doses may be necessary in some cases.

Metformin:

Ozempic can be used in combination with metformin, and this combination is often prescribed as part of the overall diabetes management plan. The complementary mechanisms of action contribute to improved glycemic control. Providers should monitor for potential gastrointestinal symptoms, and adjustments in metformin doses may be necessary.

Thiazolidinediones:

Ozempic can be used with thiazolidinediones (TZDs) when additional glycemic control is required. Providers should monitor for potential additive effects on weight and consider adjustments in TZD doses based on individual patient response.

Interaction with Drugs Affecting Renal Function:

Diuretics:

Diuretics, especially loop diuretics, may affect renal function. Ozempic, which is primarily excreted through the renal route, may require dosage adjustments in individuals using diuretics. Providers should monitor renal function and consider dosage modifications as needed.

Renin-Angiotensin-Aldosterone System (RAAS) Inhibitors:

RAAS inhibitors, such as angiotensin-converting enzyme (ACE) inhibitors and angiotensin II receptor blockers (ARBs), may impact renal function. Providers should monitor renal function closely when Ozempic is used concomitantly with RAAS inhibitors and adjust doses as necessary.

Interaction with Gastrointestinal Motility Modifying

Drugs:

Prokinetic Agents:
Prokinetic agents, which enhance gastrointestinal motility, may potentially affect the absorption and

distribution of Ozempic. Providers should monitor for changes in glycemic control and consider adjustments in Ozempic doses if necessary.

Interaction with Drugs Requiring Dosage

Adjustments:

Warfarin:

Ozempic may affect the international normalized ratio (INR) in individuals taking warfarin. Providers should closely monitor INR levels when Ozempic is initiated or doses are adjusted, and consider warfarin dosage modifications based on individual patient response.

CYP Enzyme Inducers and Inhibitors:

Ozempic undergoes metabolism primarily through cytochrome P450 (CYP) enzymes, specifically CYP2C8. Concomitant use of CYP enzyme inducers (e.g., rifampin) or inhibitors (e.g., gemfibrozil) may impact Ozempic's pharmacokinetics. Providers should be cautious and consider dosage adjustments based on individual patient responses.

Special Populations and Considerations:

Elderly Patients:

Elderly patients may be more susceptible to certain drug interactions due to age-related changes in pharmacokinetics and pharmacodynamics. Providers should carefully assess the potential risks and benefits of concomitant medications and consider dosage adjustments as needed.

Pediatric Population:

Ozempic is not indicated for use in children and adolescents, and potential drug interactions in this population are not well-established. Providers should exercise caution and consider alternative therapeutic options for pediatric patients.

Renal Impairment:

In individuals with renal impairment, dosage adjustments may be necessary for drugs that interact with Ozempic. Providers should closely monitor renal function and make appropriate adjustments to ensure the safety and efficacy of concomitant medications.

Practical Guidance for Healthcare Providers:

Comprehensive Medication Review:

Conduct a comprehensive review of the patient's current medication list, including over-the-counter and herbal supplements, before initiating Ozempic. This aids in identifying potential drug interactions and guiding treatment decisions.

Regular Monitoring:

Implement a structured monitoring plan, including regular assessments of glycemic control, renal function, and potential adverse effects. Regular follow-up appointments allow for ongoing evaluation and adjustments as needed.

Patient Education:

Thoroughly educate patients on potential drug interactions, emphasizing the importance of informing healthcare providers about all medications, including over-the-counter and herbal supplements. Patient awareness enhances collaboration in the management of diabetes.

Individualized Treatment Plans:

Individualize treatment plans based on the patient's medical history, comorbidities, and treatment goals. Consideration of potential drug interactions guides decision-making and helps optimize the overall safety and efficacy of diabetes management.

Collaboration with Specialists:

Collaborate with specialists, such as nephrologists, cardiologists, and pharmacists, when managing individuals with complex medical conditions or contraindications that require specialized expertise in drug interactions.

potential drug interactions are crucial for healthcare providers prescribing Ozempic in the management of type 2 diabetes mellitus. By considering interactions with other antidiabetic medications, drugs affecting renal function, gastrointestinal motility modifiers, and drugs requiring dosage adjustments, providers can make informed decisions to optimize the safety and efficacy of Ozempic in diverse patient populations. Regular monitoring, patient education, and collaboration with specialists contribute to a comprehensive approach in managing diabetes and mitigating potential risks associated with drug interactions.

PRECAUTIONS

Precautions play a vital role in the safe and effective use of medications, including Ozempic (semaglutide), a glucagon-like peptide-1 receptor agonist (GLP-1 RA) used in the management of type 2 diabetes mellitus. Precautions guide healthcare providers in identifying specific situations or conditions that may warrant careful consideration, monitoring, or potential adjustments when prescribing Ozempic. This extensive exploration will delve into the various precautions associated with Ozempic, covering considerations related to cardiovascular health, renal function, gastrointestinal factors, and other special populations.

Cardiovascular Precautions:

Heart Disease:

Individuals with a history of cardiovascular disease may benefit from Ozempic's cardiovascular benefits demonstrated in clinical trials. However, healthcare providers should exercise caution in patients with severe or unstable heart disease. Regular cardiovascular assessments and collaboration with cardiologists may be necessary in these cases.

Congestive Heart Failure:

Ozempic is contraindicated in individuals with a history of heart failure. In patients with a history of heart failure, or those at an increased risk, close monitoring for signs and symptoms of worsening heart failure is crucial. If heart failure develops, discontinuation of Ozempic should be considered.

Cardiovascular Risk Assessment:

Prior to initiating Ozempic, healthcare providers should assess the patient's overall cardiovascular risk. This includes evaluating factors such as a history of myocardial infarction, stroke, or peripheral vascular disease. The cardiovascular benefits observed in clinical trials may influence the decision to choose Ozempic in individuals with a high cardiovascular risk.

Renal Precautions:

Renal Impairment:

Ozempic is primarily excreted through the renal route. Providers should exercise caution in individuals with renal impairment, and dosage adjustments may be necessary in severe renal impairment or end-stage renal disease. Regular monitoring of renal function is essential.

Assessment of Renal Function:

Before initiating Ozempic, healthcare providers should assess renal function through laboratory testing, including serum creatinine and estimated glomerular filtration rate (eGFR). Periodic monitoring is recommended, especially in individuals at risk of renal impairment or those using medications that may affect renal function.

Gastrointestinal Precautions:

Gastroparesis:

Ozempic should be used with caution in individuals with gastroparesis, a condition characterized by delayed gastric emptying. Gastrointestinal symptoms associated with Ozempic, such as nausea and vomiting, may exacerbate gastroparesis. Providers should monitor for symptoms and consider alternative therapeutic options if necessary.

Inflammatory Bowel Disease (IBD):

Individuals with inflammatory bowel disease (IBD), including Crohn's disease and ulcerative colitis, may be at an increased risk of gastrointestinal adverse events with Ozempic. Providers should carefully evaluate the risks and benefits, monitor for symptoms, and consider alternative treatments if needed.

Special Populations:

Elderly Patients:

Elderly patients may be more susceptible to certain adverse effects, including gastrointestinal symptoms. Providers should carefully assess the potential risks and benefits of Ozempic in elderly individuals and consider starting at the lower end of the dosing spectrum.

Pediatric Population:

Ozempic is not indicated for use in children and adolescents. The safety and efficacy of Ozempic in the pediatric population have not been extensively studied. Providers should exercise caution and consider alternative therapeutic options for pediatric patients.

Pregnancy and Breastfeeding:

The safety of Ozempic during pregnancy and breastfeeding has not been established. Ozempic should only be used during pregnancy if the potential benefits justify the potential risks to the fetus. It is not known whether Ozempic is excreted in human breast milk.

Pancreatic Precautions:

Pancreatitis:

Pancreatitis has been reported with GLP-1 receptor agonists, including Ozempic. Providers should exercise caution in individuals with a history of pancreatitis.

Monitoring for signs and symptoms of pancreatitis, such as severe abdominal pain, is essential. Discontinuation of Ozempic should be considered if pancreatitis is suspected.

Thyroid C-Cell Tumors:

GLP-1 receptor agonists, including Ozempic, have been associated with an increased risk of thyroid C-cell tumors in animal studies. While the relevance of this finding to humans is uncertain, providers should monitor for thyroid nodules and assess thyroid function periodically.

Immunogenicity:

Antibody Formation:
As with any therapeutic protein, there is a potential for the development of antibodies to Ozempic. The clinical significance of antibody formation is not fully understood. In cases where a sustained glyccmic response is not achieved, or adverse events occur, healthcare providers may consider alternative therapeutic options.

General Precautions:

Surgery and Acute Illness:

During periods of acute illness or major surgery, the use of Ozempic may be temporarily discontinued.

Individuals may require alternative means of glycemic control during these situations.

Dosing Adjustments with Concomitant

Medications:

Concomitant use of medications that affect renal function or require dosage adjustments in renal impairment may necessitate modifications in the dosing regimen of Ozempic. Providers should carefully assess potential drug interactions.

Practical Guidance for Healthcare Providers:

Comprehensive Patient Assessment:

Conduct a thorough patient assessment, including medical history, family history, and a review of current medications, before initiating Ozempic. This comprehensive evaluation aids in identifying precautions and potential risks.

Regular Monitoring:

Implement a structured monitoring plan, including regular assessments of glycemic control, cardiovascular risk factors, renal function, and potential adverse effects. Regular follow-up appointments allow for ongoing evaluation and adjustments as needed.

Patient Education:

Thoroughly educate patients on precautions associated with Ozempic, emphasizing the importance of reporting any signs or symptoms of adverse events. Patient awareness enhances collaboration in the management of diabetes.

Individualized Treatment Plans:

Individualize treatment plans based on the patient's medical history, comorbidities, and treatment goals. Consideration of precautions guides decision-making and helps optimize the overall safety and efficacy of diabetes management.

Collaboration with Specialists:

Collaborate with specialists, such as endocrinologists, cardiologists, and nephrologists, when managing individuals with complex medical conditions or precautions that require specialized expertise.

 precautions associated with Ozempic are essential considerations for healthcare providers prescribing this GLP-1 receptor agonist in the management of type 2 diabetes mellitus. By carefully assessing cardiovascular health, renal function, gastrointestinal factors, and other special populations, providers can navigate potential risks and tailor treatment plans to individual patient needs. Regular monitoring, patient education, and collaboration with specialists contribute to a comprehensive approach in managing diabetes and mitigating potential risks associated with precautions.

CLINICAL STUDIES

Clinical studies are fundamental components of the drug development process, providing critical insights into the safety, efficacy, and overall therapeutic profile of medications. In the case of Ozempic (semaglutide), a glucagon-like peptide-1 receptor agonist (GLP-1 RA) used in the management of type 2 diabetes mellitus, a series of clinical trials have been conducted to evaluate its performance and establish its role in diabetes care. This extensive exploration will delve into key clinical studies related to Ozempic, covering its development phases, major trials, and notable findings that have contributed to its regulatory approval and adoption in clinical practice.

Ozempic:
Ozempic, also known by its generic name semaglutide, belongs to the class of GLP-1 receptor agonists. These medications mimic the effects of the endogenous incretin hormone GLP-1, enhancing insulin secretion, suppressing glucagon release, and slowing gastric emptying. Ozempic is administered subcutaneously and has demonstrated efficacy in improving glycemic control, reducing body weight, and, importantly, exhibiting cardiovascular benefits.

Development Phases:

Preclinical Studies:

Preclinical studies involving in vitro and animal experiments laid the foundation for Ozempic's development. These studies assessed the compound's pharmacokinetics, pharmacodynamics, and general safety profile. Key considerations included its impact on glucose metabolism, potential side effects, and overall tolerability.

Phase 1 Clinical Trials:

Phase 1 trials in humans focused on evaluating the safety, tolerability, and pharmacokinetics of Ozempic. These studies involved healthy volunteers and provided initial insights into its potential therapeutic use in humans. Dosage escalation and initial assessments of adverse events guided subsequent phases.

Phase 2 Clinical Trials:

Phase 2 trials expanded the investigation to individuals with type 2 diabetes. The primary goals included assessing Ozempic's efficacy in glycemic control, exploring dosage regimens, and gathering preliminary data on safety. These trials set the stage for larger-scale efficacy and safety assessments in later phases.

Phase 3 Clinical Trials:

The pivotal phase 3 trials are crucial for establishing the efficacy and safety of Ozempic in diverse patient populations. These multicenter, randomized, controlled trials involve a larger patient cohort and compare Ozempic against placebo or other antidiabetic medications. Phase 3 trials typically include assessments of glycemic control, body weight, and cardiovascular outcomes.

Key Clinical Trials:

SUSTAIN Program:

The SUSTAIN (Semaglutide Unabated Sustainability in Treatment of Type 2 Diabetes) program represents a series of phase 3 trials evaluating Ozempic's efficacy and safety. Notable trials within the SUSTAIN program include:

SUSTAIN-6: This cardiovascular outcomes trial demonstrated a significant reduction in major adverse cardiovascular events with Ozempic compared to placebo. The trial included individuals with type 2 diabetes and established cardiovascular disease or at high cardiovascular risk.

SUSTAIN-7: Focusing on glycemic control and weight reduction, SUSTAIN-7 compared Ozempic with sitagliptin, a dipeptidyl peptidase-4 (DPP-4) inhibitor. Ozempic showed superior efficacy in lowering HbA1c and body weight.

SUSTAIN-9: This trial evaluated Ozempic's efficacy and safety in individuals with type 2 diabetes and moderate renal impairment. Ozempic demonstrated sustained glycemic control and a favorable safety profile in this population.

PIONEER Program:

The PIONEER (Peptide InnOvatioN for Early diabEtes tReatment) program explored Ozempic's use in early diabetes treatment. Key trials include:
PIONEER-6: A cardiovascular outcomes trial comparing Ozempic with placebo in individuals with type 2 diabetes and established cardiovascular disease or at high cardiovascular risk. Ozempic demonstrated cardiovascular safety and reduced the risk of major adverse cardiovascular events.

PIONEER-1: Focusing on treatment-naive patients, PIONEER-1 assessed Ozempic's efficacy in reducing HbA1c compared to placebo. Ozempic exhibited significant improvements in glycemic control.

OTHER Trials:

Various other trials have explored Ozempic in specific contexts, such as:
Delivering Early Diabetes Remission (DETECT-2): Investigating the potential of Ozempic in achieving diabetes remission in individuals recently diagnosed with type 2 diabetes.

Semaglutide and Cardiovascular Outcomes in Patients with Type 2 Diabetes (SOUL): A trial assessing cardiovascular outcomes and safety in individuals with type 2 diabetes and established cardiovascular disease.

Notable Findings and Contributions:

Cardiovascular Benefits:

The SUSTAIN-6 trial was pivotal in establishing Ozempic's cardiovascular benefits. The reduction in major adverse cardiovascular events, including cardiovascular death, non-fatal myocardial infarction, and non-fatal stroke, positioned Ozempic as a valuable option for individuals with diabetes and cardiovascular comorbidities.

Glycemic Control and Weight Reduction:

Across multiple trials, Ozempic consistently demonstrated superior efficacy in improving glycemic control compared to placebo and other antidiabetic medications. Additionally, Ozempic's association with weight reduction was a significant finding, addressing a common concern in diabetes management.

Renal Safety:

The SUSTAIN-9 trial specifically addressed Ozempic's safety and efficacy in individuals with moderate renal impairment. The findings supported the use of Ozempic in this population, expanding its applicability to individuals with varying degrees of renal function.

Early Diabetes Treatment:

The PIONEER program investigated Ozempic's role in early diabetes treatment, providing valuable insights into its efficacy and safety in treatment-naive patients. This research has implications for the initiation of GLP-1 receptor agonists in the early stages of diabetes.

Regulatory Approvals:
Based on the robust evidence generated from these clinical trials, Ozempic received regulatory approvals for the treatment of type 2 diabetes in various countries. These approvals were based on the medication's demonstrated efficacy in improving glycemic control, cardiovascular safety, and its favorable side effect profile.

Ongoing Research:
The field of diabetes management is dynamic, and ongoing research continues to explore Ozempic's role in various contexts. Clinical studies may focus on long-term outcomes, real-world effectiveness, and its use in specific patient populations, contributing to the evolving landscape of diabetes care.

Practical Implications for Healthcare Providers:

Individualized Treatment Plans:

Clinical studies provide evidence supporting the efficacy and safety of Ozempic, but healthcare providers must individualize treatment plans based on patient characteristics, preferences, and comorbidities. A thorough understanding of clinical trial findings guides personalized decision-making.

Cardiovascular Assessment:

For individuals with type 2 diabetes and cardiovascular comorbidities, Ozempic's cardiovascular benefits, as demonstrated in trials like SUSTAIN-6, make it a compelling option. Cardiovascular assessments and considerations are integral in tailoring treatment plans.

PATIENT COUNSELING

Patient counseling is a crucial aspect of healthcare, fostering effective communication between healthcare providers and individuals receiving medical care. In the context of Ozempic (semaglutide), a glucagon-like peptide-1 receptor agonist (GLP-1 RA) used in the management of type 2 diabetes mellitus, counseling plays a pivotal role in ensuring optimal treatment outcomes. This extensive exploration will delve into the key components of patient counseling for Ozempic, covering aspects such as medication administration, potential side effects, lifestyle considerations, and the importance of ongoing communication between healthcare providers and patients.

Patient Counseling for Ozempic:
Patient counseling for Ozempic encompasses a comprehensive set of discussions and guidance aimed at empowering individuals with type 2 diabetes to actively participate in their treatment plan. The primary goals include enhancing patient understanding of Ozempic, promoting medication adherence, addressing potential concerns, and fostering a collaborative approach to diabetes management.

Medication Administration:

Injection Technique:

Subcutaneous Administration: Ozempic is administered subcutaneously, typically in the abdomen. Healthcare providers should demonstrate and instruct patients on proper injection technique, emphasizing the use of a rotating injection site to minimize the risk of lipodystrophy or injection site reactions.

Needle Size and Pen Usage: Patient counseling should include information on the needle size provided with the Ozempic pen, as well as the correct handling and storage of the pen. The proper use of the pen, including dosage adjustments, loading, and priming, should be clearly explained.

Injection Timing: Ozempic is often administered once weekly. Providers should guide patients on selecting a consistent day and time for injections. This fosters a routine, helping patients integrate Ozempic into their lifestyle.

Missed Doses:

In cases where a dose is missed, patients should be advised on the appropriate actions to take. Generally, if a dose is missed within five days of the scheduled injection day, it should be administered as soon as possible. If more than five days have passed, the patient should wait until the next scheduled dose.

Storage:

Proper storage of Ozempic pens is essential for maintaining medication efficacy. Patients should be informed about storing the pen in the refrigerator but not freezing it. Once in use, the pen can be kept at room temperature for a limited time. Detailed guidance on storage conditions ensures the stability of the medication.

Understanding the Medication:

Mechanism of Action:

Patient counseling should include an explanation of how Ozempic works. As a GLP-1 receptor agonist, Ozempic stimulates insulin release, suppresses glucagon secretion, and slows gastric emptying. This understanding helps patients appreciate the medication's role in managing blood glucose levels.

Benefits and Goals of Treatment:

Providers should discuss the potential benefits of Ozempic, such as improved glycemic control, weight loss, and cardiovascular benefits. Establishing realistic treatment goals in collaboration with the patient ensures a shared understanding of the desired outcomes.

Duration of Treatment:

Patients should be informed that Ozempic is typically used as a long-term treatment for type 2 diabetes.

Continuous use is essential to sustain its benefits. Discussions about treatment duration contribute to patient expectations and commitment.

Managing Potential Side Effects:

Gastrointestinal Effects:

Nausea is a common side effect of Ozempic, particularly during the initial weeks of treatment. Patient counseling should address strategies to manage nausea, such as taking Ozempic with meals. Providers should reassure patients that nausea often improves over time.

Hypoglycemia:

While Ozempic has a low risk of causing hypoglycemia when used as a monotherapy, patient counseling should emphasize the importance of regular blood glucose monitoring. In cases of concurrent use with other antidiabetic medications, patients should be educated about potential hypoglycemic risks.

Injection Site Reactions:

Patients should be informed about the possibility of injection site reactions, such as redness, swelling, or itching. These reactions are generally mild and transient. Proper injection technique, including site rotation, can help minimize these effects.

Pancreatitis and Thyroid C-Cell Tumors:

Although rare, counseling should include information on the potential risk of pancreatitis and thyroid C-cell tumors. Patients should be educated on recognizing signs and symptoms that warrant prompt medical attention.

Lifestyle Considerations:

Diet and Exercise:

Patient counseling should stress the importance of maintaining a healthy diet and engaging in regular physical activity alongside Ozempic therapy. Lifestyle modifications contribute to improved glycemic control and overall well-being.

Alcohol Consumption:

Patients should be advised about potential interactions between alcohol and Ozempic, which may increase the risk of hypoglycemia. Moderation in alcohol consumption and awareness of its effects on blood sugar levels are essential.

Weight Management:

Counseling should address the potential for weight loss with Ozempic. Patients should be encouraged to maintain a balanced approach to weight management, incorporating healthy dietary choices and regular physical activity.

Monitoring and Follow-Up:

Blood Glucose Monitoring:

Regular blood glucose monitoring is a fundamental aspect of diabetes management. Patients should be educated on the importance of self-monitoring and how to interpret glucose levels to facilitate informed decisions.

HbA1c Monitoring:

Periodic HbA1c measurements provide a comprehensive view of long-term glycemic control. Counseling should include discussions about the target HbA1c levels and the frequency of laboratory testing.

Regular Follow-Up Appointments:

Patients should understand the necessity of regular follow-up appointments with their healthcare provider. These appointments allow for ongoing assessments, adjustments to the treatment plan, and addressing any concerns or questions.

Considerations for Special Populations:

Pregnancy and Breastfeeding:

Patient counseling should highlight the importance of discussing pregnancy plans with healthcare providers. Ozempic's safety during pregnancy and breastfeeding is not well-established, and alternative therapeutic options may be considered.

Elderly Population:

Special considerations for the elderly population may include discussions about potential side effects, dosing adjustments, and the impact of comorbidities on diabetes management.

Pediatric Population:

Ozempic is not indicated for use in children and adolescents. Patient counseling for parents should emphasize alternative treatment options for pediatric patients with type 2 diabetes.

Practical Guidance for Healthcare Providers:

Patient-Centered Approach:

Adopt a patient-centered approach to counseling, considering individual preferences, lifestyle, and cultural factors. Engage in shared decision-making to establish treatment goals that align with the patient's priorities.

Clear and Understandable Language:

Use clear and understandable language during counseling sessions. Avoid medical jargon and encourage patients to ask questions for clarification.

Addressing Concerns:

Actively inquire about any concerns or reservations the patient may have. Addressing concerns promptly fosters a sense of trust and collaboration in the patient-provider relationship.

Educational Resources:

Provide written educational resources, such as pamphlets or digital materials, to reinforce key information. These resources serve as valuable references for patients to

STORAGE AND HANDLING

Storage and handling of medications, including Ozempic (semaglutide), play a crucial role in ensuring their efficacy, safety, and overall therapeutic success. Proper storage and handling procedures are essential for maintaining the stability of Ozempic, a glucagon-like peptide-1 receptor agonist (GLP-1 RA) used in the management of type 2 diabetes mellitus. This comprehensive exploration will delve into the key aspects of storing and handling Ozempic, covering topics such as storage conditions, shelf life, transportation considerations, and steps to take in case of deviations from recommended storage conditions.

Importance of Proper Storage and Handling:
Maintaining the integrity of medications is integral to their effectiveness and safety. Improper storage and handling can compromise the stability of pharmaceutical compounds, potentially leading to diminished therapeutic outcomes, altered pharmacokinetics, and increased risks of adverse events. In the case of Ozempic, adherence to recommended storage guidelines is essential to ensure its continued efficacy in managing blood glucose levels in individuals with type 2 diabetes.

Storage Conditions for Ozempic:

Refrigeration:

Ozempic should be stored in the refrigerator at a temperature between 36°F to 46°F (2°C to 8°C). Refrigeration helps preserve the stability of the medication and prevents degradation of its active ingredient, semaglutide.

Avoid Freezing:

Freezing should be strictly avoided. Ozempic should not be stored in the freezer, as freezing temperatures can lead to irreversible damage to the medication. Patients should be educated on the importance of checking for any signs of freezing, such as ice crystals, in the solution before use.

Protection from Light:

The Ozempic pen should be kept in its original carton to protect it from light. Exposure to light, especially sunlight or artificial light, can potentially degrade the medication. Storing the pen in its carton provides an additional layer of protection.

Original Packaging:

Ozempic pens should be stored in their original packaging until use. This not only protects the medication from light exposure but also helps maintain a controlled environment, reducing the risk of temperature fluctuations.

Keep Out of Reach of Children:

Like all medications, Ozempic should be kept out of reach of children. The safety features of the Ozempic pen, including the removable needle and dose display, should be emphasized to prevent accidental exposure.

Shelf Life and Expiry:

Expiration Date:

Each Ozempic pen has an expiration date printed on the packaging. Patients should be advised to check this date before using the medication. Expired medications may not provide the intended therapeutic effects and could potentially pose risks.

Discarding Expired Medication:

Patients should be instructed to properly dispose of expired Ozempic pens. Medication take-back programs or local disposal guidelines should be followed to ensure the safe and environmentally responsible disposal of expired medications.

Transportation Considerations:

Maintaining Cold Chain:

During transportation from the pharmacy to the patient's home, or in situations where the medication needs to be transported for travel, maintaining the cold chain is crucial. Portable coolers or insulated bags with ice packs can help preserve the required temperature range.

Avoiding Exposure to Extreme Temperatures:

Ozempic pens should not be exposed to extreme temperatures during transportation. Avoid leaving the medication in a car during hot or cold weather, as this can impact its stability. Patients should be advised to plan accordingly, especially during travel.

Steps in Case of Deviations:

Temperature Deviations:

In case of unintended temperature deviations, patients should contact their healthcare provider or pharmacist for guidance. Temperature-sensitive medications like Ozempic are susceptible to degradation if exposed to temperatures outside the recommended range.

Freezing Events:

If a patient suspects that Ozempic may have frozen, they should not use the medication. Instead, they should contact their healthcare provider or pharmacist for further instructions. Using frozen Ozempic can compromise its effectiveness and safety.

Visible Changes:

Patients should be educated to visually inspect Ozempic before use. If there are any visible particles, discoloration, or other changes in the solution, they should refrain from using the medication and consult their healthcare provider or pharmacist.

Expired Medication:

Patients should not use Ozempic beyond its expiration date. If they discover an expired pen, it should be safely disposed of according to local guidelines. They should contact their healthcare provider for a replacement prescription.

Special Considerations:

Traveling with Ozempic:

Patients who travel with Ozempic should plan ahead to ensure the medication remains within the recommended temperature range. Portable coolers or insulated bags can be useful, and patients should be aware of local regulations regarding the transportation of medications.

Switching from Refrigerated to Room Temperature

Storage:

Some Ozempic pens, once in use, can be stored at room temperature (below 86°F or 30°C) for up to 56 days. Patients should be instructed on the transition process and the need to discard the pen if it exceeds the allowed room temperature storage duration.

Practical Guidance for Healthcare Providers:

Educational Resources:

Provide patients with written educational resources that detail the proper storage and handling of Ozempic. Clear instructions and visual aids can enhance patient understanding.

Regular Follow-Up:

During follow-up appointments, healthcare providers should inquire about any challenges or concerns related to storage and handling. Addressing issues promptly contributes to patient confidence in managing their medication.

Integration into Lifestyle:

Assist patients in integrating the storage and handling of Ozempic into their daily routines. Discuss strategies for travel, especially when planning trips that involve variations in temperature.

Emergency Preparedness:

In emergency situations, such as power outages or natural disasters, patients should have a plan in place to safeguard their medications. This may include having a cooler with ice packs or other contingency measures.

Collaboration with Pharmacists:

Encourage patients to consult with pharmacists if they have specific questions or encounter challenges related to the storage and handling of Ozempic. Pharmacists can provide valuable guidance and address patient concerns.

Proper storage and handling of Ozempic are critical components of its successful use in the management of type 2 diabetes mellitus. Patients who are well-informed about the importance of refrigeration, protection from light, and other storage considerations are better equipped to maintain the efficacy and safety of this medication. Healthcare providers play a pivotal role in educating patients, addressing concerns, and ensuring that Ozempic is stored and handled in accordance with recommended guidelines, ultimately contributing to optimal treatment outcomes.

AVAILABILITY AND PRICING

The availability and pricing of medications are integral aspects of healthcare, influencing accessibility and affordability for individuals seeking treatment. In the case of Ozempic (semaglutide), a glucagon-like peptide-1 receptor agonist (GLP-1 RA) used in the management of type 2 diabetes mellitus, an in-depth exploration into its availability across regions and the factors influencing pricing is essential. This comprehensive analysis will delve into the global availability of Ozempic, considerations related to its accessibility, factors influencing pricing, patient assistance programs, and the broader landscape of pharmaceutical pricing and reimbursement.

Global Availability of Ozempic:
Ozempic, developed by Novo Nordisk, has seen widespread availability across various regions globally. Its regulatory approvals in numerous countries highlight its acceptance and adoption in diverse healthcare systems. The availability of Ozempic in different regions is influenced by the regulatory processes, market demands, and strategic decisions made by the manufacturer.

Regulatory Approvals:

The regulatory landscape significantly impacts the availability of Ozempic. The medication has undergone rigorous evaluations by regulatory agencies in different countries to ensure its safety, efficacy, and quality standards. Regulatory approvals, such as those from the U.S. Food and Drug Administration (FDA), the European Medicines Agency (EMA), and other national health authorities, are pivotal in allowing Ozempic to be marketed and prescribed.

Global Marketing Strategy:

Novo Nordisk, as the manufacturer of Ozempic, plays a key role in its global distribution. The company's marketing strategy and commercial agreements influence the presence of Ozempic in various markets. Collaborations with local distributors, healthcare providers, and pharmacies contribute to the medication's availability.

Market Demand and Prescribing Patterns:

The prevalence of type 2 diabetes and the specific prescribing patterns in different regions also impact the availability of Ozempic. Markets with a higher prevalence of diabetes and a strong inclination towards GLP-1 RAs may see broader accessibility to Ozempic.

Factors Influencing Pricing:
Pharmaceutical pricing is a complex interplay of various factors, ranging from research and development costs to

market competition. Understanding the factors that influence the pricing of Ozempic provides insights into the economic considerations surrounding this medication.

Research and Development Costs:

The costs associated with the research and development (R&D) of Ozempic, including preclinical studies, clinical trials, and regulatory submissions, contribute significantly to its pricing. The extensive investment in bringing a new medication to market is reflected in its pricing to recover development expenses.

Manufacturing and Quality Control:

The manufacturing processes and quality control measures for Ozempic influence its pricing. Ensuring consistent quality, adherence to regulatory standards, and the use of advanced production technologies contribute to the overall cost structure.

Market Competition:

The presence of other medications in the same therapeutic class can impact the pricing of Ozempic. Competition within the GLP-1 RA market may lead to pricing strategies aimed at gaining market share or differentiating Ozempic from other available options.

Reimbursement and Market Access Agreements:

Negotiations with payers and reimbursement policies influence the pricing strategy. Agreements with healthcare systems, insurers, and reimbursement mechanisms can affect the actual out-of-pocket costs for patients, making Ozempic more or less affordable depending on the market.

Patient Assistance Programs:

The manufacturer, Novo Nordisk, may implement patient assistance programs to enhance accessibility for individuals facing financial challenges. These programs can include discounts, co-pay assistance, or other initiatives to alleviate the financial burden on patients.

Health Economic Considerations:

Health economic assessments, including cost-effectiveness and budget impact analyses, may play a role in pricing decisions. Demonstrating the value of Ozempic in terms of improved health outcomes and potential cost savings in diabetes management can impact its pricing.

Patient Assistance Programs:
Patient assistance programs are initiatives implemented by pharmaceutical manufacturers to support individuals in accessing their medications, particularly in cases where financial constraints may limit affordability. These programs aim to reduce out-of-pocket costs,

enhance adherence, and improve overall patient outcomes.

Co-pay Assistance Programs:

Novo Nordisk may offer co-pay assistance programs for Ozempic, providing financial support to eligible patients to reduce their out-of-pocket expenses. These programs often involve the manufacturer covering a portion of the medication cost, making it more affordable for patients.

Patient Savings Cards:

Savings cards issued by the manufacturer can be presented at pharmacies to access discounts on Ozempic prescriptions. These cards may be part of patient assistance programs designed to make the medication more accessible.

Patient Assistance Foundations:

Some pharmaceutical companies collaborate with independent patient assistance foundations to extend support to individuals facing financial difficulties. These foundations may offer grants or other forms of financial assistance to eligible patients.

Government Assistance Programs:

In certain regions, government-sponsored assistance programs may exist to support individuals with diabetes in accessing necessary medications. Patients may be eligible for subsidies or other forms of financial aid.

Broader Landscape of Pharmaceutical Pricing and Reimbursement:

Market Access Challenges:

Despite global availability, some regions may face challenges in providing broad market access to Ozempic. Factors such as healthcare infrastructure, reimbursement policies, and local regulatory processes can impact the speed and extent of access.

Healthcare System Variations:

The diversity of healthcare systems globally introduces variations in pricing and reimbursement strategies. Some countries may negotiate directly with manufacturers, while others rely on market forces to determine pricing. These variations contribute to the complexity of the pharmaceutical pricing landscape.

Biosimilar Competition:

The introduction of biosimilar products in the GLP-1 RA market can influence pricing dynamics. Biosimilars, if available, may exert downward pressure on prices, potentially benefiting patients and healthcare systems.

Government Negotiations and Price Controls:

Some countries negotiate directly with pharmaceutical manufacturers to establish pricing agreements. Additionally, certain regions implement price controls to manage healthcare costs and ensure affordability. These measures can impact the pricing of medications like Ozempic.

Insurance Formulary Placement:

The placement of Ozempic on insurance formularies can affect patient access and out-of-pocket costs. Insurers negotiate with manufacturers to include specific medications on their formularies, influencing accessibility and affordability for patients.

Practical Guidance for Patients:

Insurance Coverage Verification:

Patients are encouraged to verify their insurance coverage for Ozempic. Understanding the details of their insurance plan, including co-payments, deductibles, and coverage limits, can help manage out-of-pocket costs.

Patient Assistance Programs:

Individuals experiencing financial challenges should explore patient assistance programs offered by Novo Nordisk. These programs may provide significant cost savings, making Ozempic more affordable.

Pharmacy Discounts and Generic Alternatives:

Patients can inquire about pharmacy discounts, savings cards, or generic alternatives that may offer cost-effective options for Ozempic. Discussing these options with healthcare providers or pharmacists can provide insights into affordability.

Healthcare Provider Communication:

Open communication with healthcare providers is crucial. Patients should discuss any financial concerns related to Ozempic openly.

FREQUENTLY ASKED QUESTIONS (FAQs)

What is Ozempic, and how does it work?

Ozempic is a glucagon-like peptide-1 receptor agonist (GLP-1 RA) used in the management of type 2 diabetes. It works by mimicking the effects of the incretin hormone GLP-1, promoting insulin release, suppressing glucagon secretion, and slowing gastric emptying, leading to improved blood glucose control.

How is Ozempic administered?

Ozempic is administered subcutaneously (under the skin) using a pre-filled pen. It is typically injected once a week. Healthcare providers guide patients on the proper injection technique, site rotation, and dosage adjustments.

What are the common side effects of Ozempic?

Common side effects may include nausea, vomiting, diarrhea, abdominal pain, and injection site reactions. These side effects often diminish over time. Serious but rare side effects include pancreatitis and thyroid C-cell tumors.

Does Ozempic cause weight loss?

Yes, Ozempic has been associated with weight loss. It can contribute to reduced body weight in individuals with type 2 diabetes, making it a favorable option for those seeking weight management benefits.

Can Ozempic be used with other diabetes medications?

Ozempic can be used as monotherapy or in combination with other antidiabetic medications, such as metformin or sulfonylureas. Healthcare providers tailor treatment plans based on individual patient needs.

Is Ozempic suitable for all individuals with type 2 diabetes?

Ozempic is generally indicated for adults with type 2 diabetes. However, its use may be contraindicated in certain populations, such as those with a history of pancreatitis, severe gastrointestinal disease, or hypersensitivity to semaglutide.

Can Ozempic be used during pregnancy or breastfeeding?

The safety of Ozempic during pregnancy and breastfeeding is not well-established. Pregnant or breastfeeding individuals should consult with their healthcare providers to explore alternative treatment options.

How should Ozempic be stored?

Ozempic should be stored in the refrigerator at a temperature between 36°F to 46°F (2°C to 8°C). It should not be frozen. Once in use, a pen can be stored at room temperature (below 86°F or 30°C) for up to 56 days.

What should I do if I miss a dose of Ozempic?

If a dose is missed within five days of the scheduled injection day, it should be administered as soon as possible. If more than five days have passed, patients should wait until the next scheduled dose and contact their healthcare provider.

Are there patient assistance programs for Ozempic?

Yes, Novo Nordisk, the manufacturer of Ozempic, offers patient assistance programs, including co-pay assistance and savings cards. These programs aim to make Ozempic more affordable for eligible patients.

www.ingramcontent.com/pod-product-compliance
Lightning Source LLC
Chambersburg PA
CBHW071210290526
45796CB00008B/201